The Total Diabetes Rules:

Diabetes guide, how to live with, cure and minimize your diabetes and how to prevent diabetes

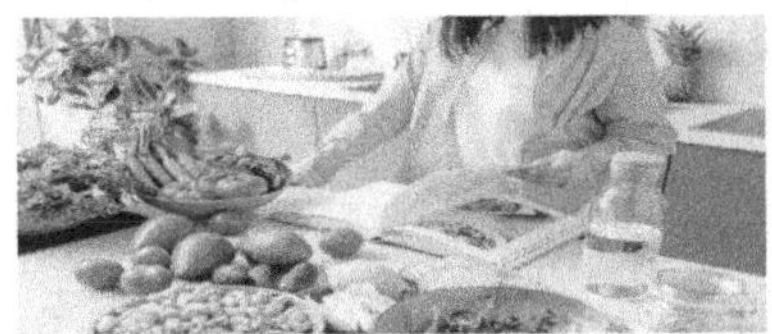

By

Flora S. Trevino

Copyright

The Total Diabetes Rules:

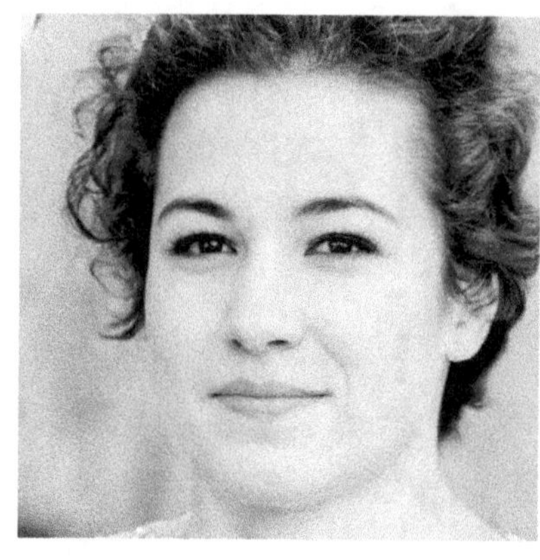

ABOUT THE AUTHOR

Meet Dr. Flora S. Trevino: Your Trusted Guide in Diabetes Care!**

With a Ph.D. in Endocrinology from Johns Hopkins University, Dr. Trevino is a distinguished expert in diabetes management.

With over 20 years of hands-on experience as a leading Endocrinologist at the esteemed MedHealth Clinic, she's transformed countless lives through her innovative approaches to diabetes care.

Dr. Trevino's passion for educating and empowering individuals shines through in her groundbreaking book, "The Total Diabetes Rules." Her comprehensive insights and practical guidance are reshaping the way we approach diabetes management!

The Total Diabetes Rules:

●

Introduction: Embracing Total Diabetes Management
9

Type 2 Diabetes: Dispelling the myths   12

Chapter 1: Understanding Diabetes   17

Introduction to Diabetes: Explaining the different
types of diabetes and their impact on the body: 17

Causes and Risk Factors:** Discussing the various
factors contributing to the development of diabetes:
21

Symptoms and Diagnosis:** Highlighting common
signs and methods for diagnosing diabetes: 26

Chapter 2: Managing Diabetes Through Diet   31

Balanced Diet Principles:** Outlining the importance
of a balanced diet in managing blood sugar levels:
31

Carbohydrates and Glycemic Index:** Explaining the
impact of carbohydrates and how to manage them
using the glycemic index: 37

Meal Planning:** Offering guidance on meal
planning, portion control, and understanding food
labels: 42

Chapter 3: Exercise and Diabetes Control   48

Benefits of Exercise:** Discussing how physical
activity aids in managing diabetes and improving
overall health: 48

Types of Exercise:** Exploring various types of
exercises suitable for individuals with diabetes: 54

Creating an Exercise Plan:** Providing a guide to
developing a personalized exercise routine.:   60

Chapter 4: Medication and Treatment   67

Understanding Medications:** Explaining different types of diabetes medications and their roles.   67

Insulin Therapy:** Detailing insulin use, administration, and its importance in diabetes management: 72

Other Treatment Options:** Highlighting alternative treatments and therapies available for diabetes.:   77

Chapter 5: Monitoring Blood Sugar Levels   84

Blood Glucose Monitoring:** Explaining the importance of regular monitoring and interpreting blood glucose readings.   84

Continuous Glucose Monitoring (CGM):** Introducing CGM devices and their benefits in diabetes management: 89

Tips for Effective Monitoring:** Providing practical tips for accurate blood sugar monitoring: 94

Chapter 6: Coping with Diabetes - Emotional Well-being   100

Managing Stress:** Discussing the impact of stress on blood sugar levels and strategies to manage stress effectively.   100

Support Systems:** Highlighting the importance of a support network and seeking professional help when needed: 106

Embracing a Positive Mindset:** Encouraging a positive attitude towards living with diabetes: 111

Chapter 7: Preventing Complications and Future Outlook   116

Complications of Diabetes:** Addressing potential complications and ways to prevent or manage them.   116

Living a Fulfilling Life:** Offering guidance on

leading a fulfilling life while managing diabetes: 122

Future of Diabetes Management:** Exploring advancements and potential breakthroughs in diabetes treatment: 127

Conclusion:Empowering Diabetes Management 132

Encouragement and Motivation:** Inspiring readers to take charge of their health and diabetes management: 137

●

Introduction: Embracing Total Diabetes Management

Welcome to "The Total Diabetes Rules."

Living with diabetes is not just about managing blood sugar levels; it's a comprehensive journey that encompasses various aspects of life. Whether you've recently been diagnosed or have been navigating this condition for some time, this book aims to be your guide, your companion, and your source of empowerment on this journey.

Understanding Diabetes as a Lifestyle

Diabetes is more than a medical condition; it's a lifestyle that requires careful attention to diet, exercise, medication, emotional well-being, and more. It's about making informed choices every day to manage your health effectively.

Empowering You with Knowledge

"The Total Diabetes Rules" isn't just about rules; it's a comprehensive approach designed to equip you with the knowledge, strategies, and motivation to live life to the fullest while managing diabetes effectively.

What You'll Find in This Book

This book is structured to cover various facets of diabetes management, from understanding the condition and its impact on your body to practical tips on diet, exercise, medication, and emotional well-being. It's a holistic guide that aims to provide actionable advice tailored to your daily life.

Your Partner in the Journey

Consider this book your partner – here to inform, support, and guide you through the intricacies of diabetes management. It's a resource crafted to empower you to take charge of your health, make informed decisions, and embrace a fulfilling life despite the challenges diabetes may present.

Let's Begin the Journey Together

Embark on this journey with an open mind, a willingness to learn, and the determination to implement positive changes. By integrating the principles outlined in this book into your daily routine, you'll discover that managing diabetes isn't just about adhering to rules; it's about embracing a lifestyle that promotes well-being and resilience.

Welcome to "The Total Diabetes Rules." Let's navigate this path together towards a healthier and happier life.

Type 2 Diabetes: Dispelling the myths

Absolutely, there are several common myths surrounding Type 2 diabetes. Let's debunk some of them:

Myth 1: Diabetes only affects people who are overweight.
- Fact: While excess weight can increase the risk of Type 2 diabetes, it's not the sole factor. Genetics, family history, poor diet, lack of physical activity, and other factors also contribute to its development.

Myth 2: People with diabetes can't eat sugar.
- Fact: Individuals with diabetes can consume sugar in moderation as part of a balanced diet. The key is moderation and monitoring carbohydrate intake rather than completely avoiding sugar.

Myth 3: Diabetes is brought about by eating an excessive amount of sugar.
- Fact: Sugar intake is not the sole cause of Type 2 diabetes. It's influenced by various factors like genetics, lifestyle, and overall diet quality.

Myth 4: Diabetes is definitely not a difficult condition.
- Fact: Diabetes can lead to severe complications if not managed properly. It can result in heart disease, stroke, kidney failure, nerve damage, and vision problems if left untreated or poorly managed.

Myth 5: Insulin is only required for people with Type 1 diabetes.
- Fact: While Type 1 diabetes requires insulin because the body doesn't produce it, some people with Type 2 diabetes may also need insulin therapy when oral medications are not effective in controlling blood sugar levels.

Myth 6: Diabetes is contagious.
- Fact: Diabetes is certainly not an infectious sickness; it can't be communicated from one individual to another like a cold or influenza.

Myth 7: Once diagnosed with diabetes, it's not reversible.

- Fact: While diabetes is a chronic condition, lifestyle changes such as healthy eating, regular exercise, and weight management can help control blood sugar levels and, in some cases, even lead to remission.

Dispelling these myths is crucial for creating a better understanding of diabetes, promoting awareness, and encouraging individuals to adopt healthier lifestyles and effective management strategies.

Chapter 1: Understanding Diabetes

Introduction to Diabetes: Explaining the different types of diabetes and their impact on the body:

Diabetes is a chronic condition that affects how your body processes glucose, or blood sugar. Glucose is a crucial energy source for cells, and its levels are regulated by insulin, a hormone produced by the pancreas. When this process falters, it leads to various types of diabetes, each with its distinct characteristics and impact on the body.

Types of Diabetes:

1. **Type 1 Diabetes:** This type occurs when the immune system attacks and destroys insulin-producing cells in the pancreas. As a result, the body produces little to no insulin, leading to an imbalance in blood sugar levels. Type 1 diabetes often develops in children or young adults and requires lifelong insulin injections or pump use for management.

2. **Type 2 Diabetes:** The most common type, characterized by insulin resistance or the body's inability to use insulin effectively. Initially, the pancreas compensates by producing more insulin, but over time, it can't keep up, leading to high blood sugar levels. Type 2 diabetes is influenced by genetic and lifestyle factors and can be managed through diet, exercise, oral medications, or insulin injections.

3. **Gestational Diabetes:** Occurs during pregnancy when hormonal changes affect insulin's effectiveness. Though temporary, it increases the risk of complications during pregnancy and childbirth. Women with gestational diabetes are at higher risk of developing type 2 diabetes later in life.

4. **Other Types:** Some diabetes types stem from specific genetic conditions, pancreatic disease, medication side effects, or other factors affecting insulin production or function.

Impact on the Body:

- **High Blood Sugar (Hyperglycemia):** Elevated blood sugar levels can cause various symptoms like increased thirst, frequent urination, fatigue, blurred vision, and slow wound healing.

-    **Long-term   Complications:**   If unmanaged, diabetes can lead to serious health complications such as cardiovascular diseases, nerve damage, kidney dysfunction, eye problems, and foot complications.

Understanding the different types of diabetes and their impact on the body is the first step toward effective management. With proper education, lifestyle adjustments, and medical guidance, individuals can proactively manage their diabetes and reduce the risk of complications, leading to a healthier and more fulfilling life despite the challenges posed by this condition.

Causes and Risk Factors:** Discussing the various factors contributing to the development of diabetes:

The development of diabetes involves a complex interplay of genetic, lifestyle, and environmental factors. Understanding these causes and risk factors is crucial in comprehending the condition's onset and progression.

Factors Contributing to Diabetes Development:

1. **Genetics and Family History:** Having a family history of diabetes increases the likelihood of developing the condition. Genetic predisposition plays a significant role, especially in type 1 diabetes, but also influences the risk of type 2 diabetes.

2.   **Lifestyle   Factors:**   Sedentary lifestyles, poor dietary choices high in refined sugars, unhealthy fats, and processed foods contribute significantly to the risk of developing type 2 diabetes. Lack of physical activity and excessive weight gain are major contributors.

3. **Insulin Resistance:** In type 2 diabetes, cells become resistant to the effects of insulin, causing blood sugar levels to rise. This resistance is often linked to excess body weight, especially around the abdomen.

4. **Gestational Factors:** Women who experience gestational diabetes during pregnancy are at increased risk of developing type 2 diabetes later in life. Additionally, children born to mothers with gestational diabetes have a higher risk of developing diabetes.

5. **Age and Ethnicity:** Age plays a role, with type 2 diabetes being more common in older adults. Moreover, certain ethnic groups, such as African Americans, Hispanic/Latino Americans, Native Americans, Asian Americans, and Pacific Islanders, have a higher predisposition to diabetes.

6. **Medical Conditions and Medications:** Some medical conditions, like polycystic ovary syndrome (PCOS) and certain medications (e.g., corticosteroids), can increase the risk of diabetes.

Environmental Influences:

1. **Urbanization and Sedentary Lifestyles:** Urban environments with less physical activity and increased reliance on processed foods contribute to the rising prevalence of diabetes.

2. **Stress and Sleep Deprivation:** Chronic stress and inadequate sleep patterns may impact insulin sensitivity and contribute to diabetes risk.

Conclusion:

The development of diabetes is a multifaceted process influenced by a combination of genetic predisposition, lifestyle choices, environmental factors, and specific medical conditions. Recognizing these factors allows for targeted interventions, emphasizing the importance of healthy lifestyle modifications, regular screenings, and proactive management to reduce the risk of diabetes or its complications.

Symptoms and Diagnosis:** Highlighting common signs and methods for diagnosing diabetes:

Recognizing the symptoms and undergoing timely diagnosis are crucial in managing diabetes effectively. Here are the common signs and diagnostic methods:

Common Symptoms of Diabetes:

1. **Excessive Thirst and Urination:** Feeling excessively thirsty and needing to urinate frequently, especially at night, are early signs of diabetes.

2. **Increased Hunger:** Experiencing frequent hunger despite eating is common,

especially in individuals with uncontrolled blood sugar levels.

3. **Fatigue:** Feeling unusually tired, weak, or fatigued, even after adequate rest, can be a symptom of high blood sugar levels.

4. **Blurred Vision:** High blood sugar levels can affect the lenses of the eyes, leading to blurred vision or other vision changes.

5. **Slow Healing of Wounds:** Wounds or sores that take longer to heal than usual can be indicative of diabetes-related circulation issues.

6. **Unexplained Weight Loss:** Unintended weight loss, despite normal or increased food intake, can occur in individuals with undiagnosed diabetes.

Methods for Diagnosing Diabetes:

1. **Blood Sugar Tests:**
   - **Fasting Plasma Glucose (FPG) Test:** Measures blood sugar levels after fasting for at least eight hours.
   - **Oral Glucose Tolerance Test (OGTT):** Involves fasting and then consuming a sugary drink to measure blood sugar levels after two hours.
   - **Hemoglobin A1c Test:** Measures average blood sugar levels over the past two to three months.

2. **Symptoms and Physical Examination:** Healthcare providers evaluate symptoms, conduct physical exams, and consider risk factors to aid in diagnosis.

3. **Additional Tests:** In some cases, additional tests such as random blood sugar tests, urine tests for glucose and ketones, or

antibody tests may be recommended for a definitive diagnosis.

Importance of Early Diagnosis:

- **Early Intervention:** Timely diagnosis allows for early intervention, enabling individuals to begin proper management strategies promptly.
- **Prevention of Complications:** Early diagnosis and management help prevent or delay potential complications associated with uncontrolled diabetes.

Conclusion:

Recognizing the signs and undergoing appropriate diagnostic tests are pivotal steps in identifying diabetes at an early stage. It's essential to seek medical advice if experiencing any symptoms or if there's a family history or other risk factors for diabetes. Early diagnosis empowers individuals to initiate appropriate lifestyle changes and medical interventions for effective diabetes management.

Chapter 2: Managing Diabetes Through Diet

Balanced Diet Principles:** Outlining the importance of a balanced diet in managing blood sugar levels:

Maintaining a balanced diet is fundamental in managing blood sugar levels and overall health for individuals with diabetes. Here's why:

Importance of a Balanced Diet for Diabetes Management:

1. **Blood Sugar Control:** A balanced diet helps regulate blood sugar levels, preventing

sharp spikes or drops in glucose levels. It's crucial for managing diabetes effectively.

2. **Nutrient Intake:** Balancing macronutrients like carbohydrates, proteins, and fats, along with micronutrients like vitamins and minerals, supports overall health and vitality.

3. **Weight Management:** A balanced diet contributes to maintaining a healthy weight, crucial for managing type 2 diabetes and reducing insulin resistance.

4. **Energy Levels:** It provides a steady and consistent supply of energy, preventing fluctuations that can impact energy levels and overall well-being.

Principles of a Balanced Diet for Diabetes:

1. **Carbohydrate Management:**
   - **Complex Carbohydrates:** Emphasize whole grains, vegetables, fruits, legumes, and low-fat dairy for sustained energy and better blood sugar control.
   - **Portion Control:** Monitor portion sizes to manage carbohydrate intake and avoid sudden spikes in blood sugar levels.

2. **Protein Intake:**
   - **Lean Protein Sources:** Include lean meats, poultry, fish, eggs, nuts, seeds, and legumes to provide essential amino acids and aid in maintaining muscle mass.

3. **Healthy Fats:**
   - **Monounsaturated and Polyunsaturated Fats:** Incorporate sources like olive oil,

avocados, nuts, and seeds for heart health and satiety.

4. **Fiber-Rich Foods:**
    - **High-Fiber Choices:** Opt for fiber-rich foods like whole grains, vegetables, fruits, and legumes to aid digestion, control blood sugar, and promote fullness.

5. **Hydration:**
    - **Water Consumption:** Ensure adequate water intake to maintain hydration levels and assist in various bodily functions.

Benefits of a Balanced Diet in Diabetes Management:

1. **Stable Blood Sugar Levels:** Balancing meals helps prevent drastic fluctuations in blood sugar levels, promoting better glycemic control.

2. **Improved Weight Management:** Portion control and nutrient-dense choices support weight management, vital in type 2 diabetes.

3. **Reduced Risk of Complications:** A balanced diet lowers the risk of diabetes-related complications like heart disease, nerve damage, and kidney problems.

Conclusion:

Adopting a balanced diet comprising nutrient-rich, portion-controlled meals is a cornerstone in managing blood sugar levels and overall health for individuals with diabetes. It empowers individuals to make healthier food choices, promoting stable blood sugar levels, weight management, and a reduced risk of complications associated with diabetes.

Carbohydrates and Glycemic Index:** Explaining the impact of carbohydrates and how to manage them using the glycemic index:

Understanding carbohydrates and their impact on blood sugar levels is crucial for individuals managing diabetes. The glycemic index (GI) is a valuable tool in managing carbohydrates effectively. Here's an explanation:

Effect of Starches on Glucose Levels:

1.   **Carbohydrate Breakdown:** Carbohydrates are broken down into glucose

during digestion, causing an increase in blood sugar levels.

2. **Glycemic Response:** Different carbohydrate-containing foods affect blood sugar levels differently. Some cause rapid spikes (high glycemic foods), while others lead to slower, more controlled increases (low glycemic foods).

The Glycemic Index (GI):

1. **Definition:** The glycemic index measures how quickly a carbohydrate-containing food raises blood sugar levels compared to pure glucose (which has a GI of 100).

2. **GI Scale:**
    - **Low GI (55 or less):** Foods that produce a slower and more gradual increase in blood sugar levels.

- **Medium GI (56-69):** Foods that lead to a moderate increase in blood sugar levels.
- **High GI (70 and above):** Foods that cause a rapid spike in blood sugar levels.

Managing Carbohydrates Using the Glycemic Index:

1. **Choosing Low GI Foods:** Opt for foods with a lower GI to help control blood sugar levels more effectively. Examples include:
   - **Entire grains:** Oats, grain, quinoa, and entire wheat items.
   - **Non-starchy vegetables:** Broccoli, spinach, and carrots.
   - **Legumes:** Beans, lentils, and chickpeas.

2. **Balancing Meals:** Combine low or medium GI foods with lean protein and

healthy fats to further moderate the glycemic response.

3. **Portion Control:** Managing portion sizes of high GI foods can help mitigate their impact on blood sugar levels.

4. **Considering Other Factors:** While GI is a helpful tool, it's essential to consider other factors such as food preparation, fiber content, and individual metabolic responses to accurately manage blood sugar levels.

Benefits of Utilizing the Glycemic Index:

1. **Blood Sugar Control:** Choosing low GI foods assists in maintaining more stable blood sugar levels over time.

2. **Satiety and Weight Management:** Low GI foods tend to promote a feeling of fullness, aiding in weight management.

3. **Reduced Risk of Complications:** Incorporating low GI foods may help reduce the risk of diabetes-related complications.

Conclusion:

Understanding carbohydrates and using the glycemic index as a guide can assist individuals with diabetes in making informed food choices, managing blood sugar levels effectively, and promoting overall health. Incorporating a variety of low to medium GI foods while considering portion sizes contributes to better glycemic control and overall well-being.

Meal Planning:** Offering guidance on meal planning, portion control, and understanding food labels:

Meal planning, portion control, and understanding food labels are integral components of managing diabetes effectively. Here's guidance on incorporating these aspects into a diabetes-friendly eating routine:

Meal Planning for Diabetes:

1. **Regular Meal Schedule:** Aim for consistent meal times to regulate blood sugar levels. Include three main meals and healthy snacks if needed.

2. **Balanced Plate Method:** Divide meals to include:

- **50% Non-Starchy Vegetables:** Such as leafy greens, peppers, tomatoes, and broccoli.
    - **25% Lean Proteins:** Like poultry, fish, tofu, or legumes.
    - **25% Whole Grains or Starchy Vegetables:** Quinoa, brown rice, sweet potatoes, or whole-grain bread.

3. **Limiting Sugary Foods:** Minimize intake of sugary beverages, desserts, and processed snacks.

Portion Control:

1. **Use Measuring Tools:** Initially measure portions to understand proper serving sizes. Gradually, develop an eye for portion estimation.

2. **Plate Method or Hand Portion Control:** Use visual aids like the plate

method or your hand to estimate portion sizes.

3. **Avoid Oversized Servings:** Be mindful of restaurant portions, often larger than necessary. Consider sharing or saving part for later.

Understanding Food Labels:

1. **Reading Labels:** Check serving sizes, total carbohydrates, fiber, and added sugars.

2. **Focus on Carbohydrates:** Look for low GI and high-fiber options. Be cautious of hidden sugars and opt for whole food alternatives.

3. **Ingredient List:** Prioritize foods with fewer processed ingredients and artificial additives.

Practical Tips for Meal Planning:

1. **Preparation is Key:** Plan meals in advance, create shopping lists, and prep ingredients for the week to make healthy choices more accessible.

2. **Experiment with Recipes:** Explore healthier cooking methods and recipes tailored to diabetes-friendly ingredients.

3. **Regular Monitoring:** Monitor blood sugar levels after meals to gauge how specific foods affect individual responses.

Benefits of Meal Planning, Portion Control, and Label Understanding:

1. **Stable Blood Sugar Levels:** Controlled portions and well-planned meals aid in managing blood sugar levels.

2. **Weight Management:** Portion control supports weight maintenance or weight loss goals if necessary.

3. **Improved Nutrition:** Understanding food labels ensures intake of nutrient-dense, diabetes-friendly foods.

Conclusion:

Implementing meal planning strategies, practicing portion control, and deciphering food labels play pivotal roles in managing diabetes effectively. By incorporating these practices, individuals can create balanced, diabetes-friendly meals, regulate blood sugar levels, and improve overall health and well-being.

Chapter 3: Exercise and Diabetes Control

Benefits of Exercise:** Discussing how physical activity aids in managing diabetes and improving overall health:

Physical activity offers numerous benefits for individuals managing diabetes and contributes to overall health and well-being. Here's how exercise positively impacts diabetes management:

Benefits of Exercise for Diabetes Management:

1. **Improved Insulin Sensitivity:** Regular physical activity enhances the body's ability to use insulin effectively, thereby improving blood sugar regulation.

2. **Better Blood Sugar Control:** Exercise helps lower blood sugar levels by facilitating glucose uptake by muscles, even without additional insulin.

3. **Weight Management:** Physical activity assists in weight loss or maintenance, crucial for managing type 2 diabetes and reducing insulin resistance.

4. **Enhanced Cardiovascular Health:** Exercise strengthens the heart, lowers blood pressure, and reduces the risk of heart disease – a common complication in diabetes.

5. **Increased Muscle Strength and Endurance:** Building muscle through

exercise supports better glucose metabolism and overall physical function.

6. **Improved Mood and Stress Management:** Physical activity stimulates the release of endorphins, promoting feelings of well-being and reducing stress, which can impact blood sugar levels.

Types of Exercise Recommended for Diabetes:

1. **Aerobic Exercise:** Activities like brisk walking, jogging, cycling, swimming, and dancing improve cardiovascular health and aid in blood sugar control.

2. **Strength Training:** Using weights or resistance bands helps build muscle strength, promoting better glucose utilization.

3. **Flexibility and Balance Exercises:** Practices like yoga or tai chi enhance flexibility, balance, and overall well-being.

Exercise Guidelines for Individuals with Diabetes:

1. **Consistency:** Aim for regular exercise, aiming for at least 150 minutes of moderate-intensity aerobic exercise per week, spread across several days.

2. **Gradual Progression:** Start slowly and gradually increase intensity and duration as fitness improves.

3. **Consultation with Healthcare Providers:** Individuals with diabetes, especially those on specific medications, should consult healthcare providers before starting a new exercise regimen.

Additional Benefits of Exercise:

1. **Improved Sleep Quality:** Regular physical activity can promote better sleep patterns, contributing to overall health.

2. **Enhanced Energy Levels:** Exercise increases energy levels and reduces fatigue, improving quality of life.

Conclusion:

Incorporating regular physical activity into daily routines is a cornerstone of diabetes management. Exercise not only aids in better blood sugar control and insulin sensitivity but also promotes overall health, cardiovascular fitness, mental well-being, and energy levels for individuals managing diabetes.

Types of Exercise:** Exploring various types of exercises suitable for individuals with diabetes:

Absolutely! Here are various types of exercises suitable for individuals managing diabetes, catering to different fitness levels and preferences:

1. Aerobic Exercises:

1. **Brisk Walking:** An excellent low-impact activity that improves cardiovascular health without requiring any special equipment.

2. **Cycling:** Whether outdoors or using a stationary bike, cycling boosts heart health and aids in weight management.

3. **Swimming or Water Aerobics:** Ideal for those with joint issues as water exercises are gentle on the joints while providing a full-body workout.

4. **Dancing:** Engaging in dance classes or following dance routines improves cardiovascular fitness while being enjoyable.

2. Strength Training:

1. **Bodyweight Exercises:** Utilizing one's body weight for exercises like squats, lunges, push-ups, and planks to build muscle strength.

2. **Resistance Band Workouts:** Using resistance bands provides resistance for muscle strengthening exercises without needing heavy weights.

3. **Weight Training:** Incorporating free weights or machines at the gym to increase muscle mass and enhance metabolism.

3. Flexibility and Balance Exercises:

1. **Yoga:** Enhances flexibility, balance, and relaxation, combining physical postures with breathing exercises.

2. **Tai Chi:** A gentle martial art that improves balance, flexibility, and relaxation through slow, flowing movements.

3. **Stretching Exercises:** Engaging in stretching routines to increase flexibility and prevent muscle stiffness.

4. Interval Training:

1. **High-Intensity Interval Training (HIIT):** Alternating between short bursts of

intense exercise and periods of rest or lower intensity workouts. Powerful for working on cardiovascular wellness and consuming calories

2. **Tabata Workouts:** High-intensity intervals for short periods (20 seconds of exercise followed by 10 seconds of rest) repeated several times.

5. Daily Activities:

1. **Household Chores:** Activities like gardening, cleaning, or yard work contribute to physical activity levels.

2. **Taking the Stairs:** Opting for stairs instead of elevators or escalators incrcases daily activity levels.

Considerations:

1. **Personalization:** Choose exercises that match individual fitness levels, interests, and health conditions.

2. **Consultation:** Always consult a healthcare provider before starting a new exercise program, especially for individuals with specific health concerns or complications related to diabetes.

3. **Gradual Progression:** Start slowly and gradually increase intensity and duration to avoid injury or overexertion.

Conclusion:

Various types of exercises cater to different fitness levels and preferences, offering a range of options for individuals managing diabetes. Incorporating a combination of aerobic, strength, flexibility, and balance exercises into one's routine helps improve overall health, blood sugar control, and quality of life for those living with diabetes.

Creating an Exercise Plan:** Providing a guide to developing a personalized exercise routine.:

Certainly! Here's a guide to creating a personalized exercise plan tailored to individuals managing diabetes:

1. Set Clear Goals:

1. **Define Objectives:** Identify specific fitness goals, whether it's improving cardiovascular health, increasing muscle

strength, managing weight, or enhancing overall well-being.

2. **Establish Realistic Targets:** Set achievable and realistic short-term and long-term goals based on individual abilities and health conditions.

2. Consult Healthcare Providers:

1. **Health Assessment:** Discuss exercise plans and goals with healthcare providers or fitness professionals to ensure they align with individual health conditions and medications.

2. **Seek Guidance:** Consider consulting with a certified diabetes educator, exercise physiologist, or fitness trainer experienced in working with individuals with diabetes.

3. Choose Suitable Exercises:

1.   **Consider Preferences:** Select exercises that match personal interests, ensuring adherence to the routine.

2. **Diversify Workout:** Incorporate a combination of aerobic, strength training, flexibility, and balance exercises for a well-rounded routine.

4. Design the Exercise Plan:

1. **Frequency:** Aim for at least 150 minutes of moderate-intensity aerobic exercise spread across several days of the week, as per guidelines.

2. **Mix Exercise Types:** Schedule a variety of exercises throughout the week to engage different muscle groups and prevent monotony.

3. **Gradual Progression:** Start with manageable intensity and duration, gradually increasing as fitness levels improve.

5. Warm-Up and Cool-Down:

1. **Warm-Up:** Begin each session with 5-10 minutes of light cardio (walking, cycling) to prepare the body for exercise.

2. **Cool-Down:** End workouts with 5-10 minutes of stretching exercises to prevent muscle soreness and promote flexibility.

6. Monitor Progress:

1. **Track Workouts:** Maintain a workout journal or use fitness apps to monitor exercise sessions, noting intensity, duration, and how the body responds.

2. **Assess Adjustments:** Regularly evaluate progress towards set goals and adjust the exercise plan accordingly.

7. Address Safety Measures:

1. **Hydration:** Stay well-hydrated before, during, and after workouts.

2. **Blood Sugar Monitoring:** Check blood sugar levels before and after exercise to understand how the body responds and make necessary adjustments.

8. Consider Lifestyle Integration:

1. **Incorporate Daily Activity:** Incorporate more physical activity into daily routines, such as walking breaks, taking the stairs, or household chores.

2. **Consistency is Key:** Stick to the exercise plan consistently to yield optimal results and experience long-term benefits.

Conclusion:

Developing a personalized exercise plan involves goal-setting, choosing suitable exercises, gradual progression, monitoring progress, and considering safety measures. By designing a tailored routine aligned with individual abilities and health conditions, individuals managing diabetes can enjoy the benefits of exercise while effectively managing their health.

Chapter 4: Medication and Treatment

Understanding Medications:** Explaining different types of diabetes medications and their roles.

Of course! Diabetes medications serve various purposes in managing blood sugar levels and the condition's overall control. Here are different types of diabetes medications and their roles:

1. Insulin:

- **Role:** Regulates blood sugar levels by helping glucose enter cells for energy or storage. Different types (rapid, short, intermediate, long-acting) mimic the body's natural insulin production.

2. **Oral Medications for Type 2 Diabetes:**

- **Metformin:**
    - **Role:** Reduces liver glucose production and enhances insulin sensitivity in muscle cells, improving glucose uptake.

- **Sulfonylureas (e.g., Glipizide, Glyburide):**
    - **Role:** Stimulate the pancreas to release more insulin.

- **Meglitinides (e.g., Repaglinide, Nateglinide):**
    - **Role:** Stimulate insulin release from the pancreas, particularly after meals.

- **Thiazolidinediones (e.g., Pioglitazone, Rosiglitazone):**
  - **Role:** Increase insulin sensitivity in muscle and fat cells, reducing liver glucose production.

- **DPP-4 Inhibitors (e.g., Sitagliptin, Saxagliptin):**
  - **Role:** Enhance insulin release and inhibit glucagon release, reducing liver glucose production.

- **GLP-1 Receptor Agonists (e.g., Exenatide, Liraglutide):**
  - **Role:** Stimulate insulin secretion, slow stomach emptying, reduce glucagon secretion, and may assist with weight loss.

- **SGLT2 Inhibitors (e.g., Canagliflozin, Dapagliflozin):**

- **Role:** Block glucose reabsorption in the kidneys, increasing glucose excretion in urine.

- **Alpha-glucosidase Inhibitors (e.g., Acarbose, Miglitol):**
  - **Role:** Slow carbohydrate digestion and absorption, reducing post-meal blood sugar spikes.

Other Medications:

- **Aspirin:** Often recommended to reduce the risk of heart attack and stroke in individuals with diabetes.

- **Cholesterol-lowering Medications (Statins):** Prescribed to manage cholesterol levels and reduce the risk of cardiovascular complications in diabetes.

Conclusion:

Different diabetes medications work through various mechanisms, aiming to control blood sugar levels and reduce complications. The choice of medication depends on individual health factors, type of diabetes, and treatment goals. It's crucial to work closely with healthcare providers to determine the most suitable medication or combination of medications for optimal diabetes management.

Insulin Therapy: Detailing insulin use, administration, and its importance in diabetes management:

Certainly! Insulin therapy is a cornerstone in managing diabetes, particularly in individuals with type 1 diabetes and some with type 2 diabetes. Here's an overview of insulin therapy, its administration, and its significance in diabetes management:

Insulin in Diabetes Management:

1. **Type 1 Diabetes:** People with type 1 diabetes rely on insulin therapy as their pancreas produces little to no insulin.

2. **Type 2 Diabetes:** Some individuals with type 2 diabetes may require insulin when other medications or lifestyle changes are insufficient in controlling blood sugar levels.

Types of Insulin:

1. **Rapid-Acting Insulin:** Begins working within 15 minutes, peaks in about an hour, and lasts for 2-4 hours.

2. **Short-Acting (Regular) Insulin:** Starts working within 30 minutes, peaks in 2-3 hours, and remains active for about 3-6 hours.

3. **Intermediate-Acting Insulin:** Onset takes 2-4 hours, peaks in 4-12 hours, and lasts up to 18 hours.

4. **Long-Acting Insulin:** Slow and steady release over 24 hours, maintaining stable blood sugar levels without pronounced peaks.

Administration Methods:

1. **Insulin Injection:** Administered through syringes, insulin pens, or insulin

pumps. Injection sites typically include the abdomen, thighs, upper arms, or buttocks.

2. **Continuous Subcutaneous Insulin Infusion (CSII) - Insulin Pump:** Delivers insulin continuously through a small device connected to the body via a tube or patch.

Importance in Diabetes Management:

1. **Regulates Blood Sugar Levels:** Insulin helps glucose enter cells, reducing high blood sugar levels and preventing complications associated with hyperglycemia.

2. **Mimics Natural Insulin Production:** Provides the body with the necessary insulin it cannot produce, allowing cells to use glucose for energy.

3. **Prevents Complications:** Proper insulin management reduces the risk of diabetes-related complications such as nerve damage, eye problems, kidney disease, and cardiovascular issues.

Individualization and Monitoring:

1. **Dose Adjustment:** Insulin doses vary based on individual needs, taking into account factors like diet, exercise, stress, illness, and blood sugar levels.

2. **Regular Monitoring:** Consistent blood sugar monitoring is essential to adjust insulin doses and prevent episodes of hypoglycemia (low blood sugar) or hyperglycemia (high blood sugar).

Conclusion:

Insulin therapy plays a vital role in diabetes management, ensuring proper regulation of blood sugar levels to prevent complications. Understanding insulin types, proper administration techniques, and personalized management are crucial for effective diabetes care, leading to improved health and quality of life for individuals managing diabetes. Regular communication with healthcare providers is essential to optimize insulin therapy and overall diabetes management.

Other Treatment Options:** Highlighting alternative treatments and therapies available for diabetes.:

Certainly! In addition to traditional medications and insulin therapy, there are alternative treatment options and complementary therapies that some individuals with diabetes explore. While these approaches may not replace conventional treatments, they can complement standard care. Here are some alternative treatments and therapies:

1. Dietary Supplements:

1. **Chromium:** Thought to enhance the action of insulin and help control blood sugar levels.

2. **Alpha-Lipoic Acid:** Acts as an antioxidant and may help with nerve-related symptoms of diabetes.

3. **Cinnamon:** Some studies suggest it might help improve insulin sensitivity.

2. Herbal Remedies:

1. **Bitter Melon:** Contains compounds that may help lower blood sugar levels.

2. **Ginseng:** Some research indicates it might help improve insulin sensitivity.

3. **Fenugreek:** Contains soluble fiber and may help with blood sugar control.

3. Acupuncture:

- **Role:** Some individuals use acupuncture to manage pain, improve circulation, and potentially aid in diabetes symptom management.

4. Mind-Body Therapies:

1. **Yoga:** Can promote relaxation, reduce stress, and improve flexibility and balance.

2. **Meditation and Deep Breathing:** Techniques to manage stress, which can impact blood sugar levels.

5. Naturopathy and Homeopathy:

- **Role:** Some individuals explore these practices to manage diabetes symptoms, focusing on natural remedies and holistic approaches.

6. Physical Activity and Lifestyle Changes:

- **Regular Exercise:** Aside from medication, maintaining an active lifestyle and a healthy diet are crucial components of managing diabetes.

Important Considerations:

1. **Consultation:** Always consult healthcare providers before incorporating alternative treatments to ensure they align with existing medications and health conditions.

2. **Evidence-Based Practices:** Many alternative treatments lack extensive scientific evidence for their effectiveness in managing diabetes.

3. **Integration with Conventional Care:** Alternative treatments should complement, not replace, conventional diabetes management strategies.

Conclusion:

While some individuals may explore alternative treatments and complementary therapies to manage diabetes symptoms, it's crucial to approach them with caution, ensuring they align with professional medical advice and do not interfere with prescribed medications or traditional diabetes management plans. Integrating these approaches cautiously, under the guidance of healthcare providers, can potentially offer additional support in managing diabetes and improving overall well-being.

Chapter 5: Monitoring Blood Sugar Levels

Blood Glucose Monitoring:** Explaining the importance of regular monitoring and interpreting blood glucose readings.

Regular blood glucose monitoring is essential for individuals managing diabetes as it provides crucial insights into their condition and helps in making informed decisions about treatment and lifestyle adjustments. Here's why it's important and how to interpret blood glucose readings:

Importance of Regular Monitoring:

1. **Managing Blood Sugar Levels:** Monitoring helps individuals understand how their food choices, physical activity, medications, and other factors impact blood sugar levels.

2. **Preventing Complications:** Regular monitoring allows for early detection of fluctuations, reducing the risk of hyperglycemia (high blood sugar) or hypoglycemia (low blood sugar) and their associated complications.

3. **Treatment Adjustments:** It aids in adjusting insulin doses, medications, diet, and exercise routines based on blood sugar trends, ensuring optimal management of diabetes.

Interpreting Blood Glucose Readings:

1. **Target Ranges:** Blood sugar targets vary for individuals, but generally, before meals (fasting), readings between 80-130 mg/dL are ideal, while after meals, readings below 180 mg/dL are commonly targeted.

2. **Hyperglycemia (High Blood Sugar):**
   - **Symptoms:** Increased thirst, frequent urination, fatigue, blurred vision.
   - **Readings:** Typically above 180 mg/dL.
   - **Action:** Address high blood sugar with additional insulin or medication, increased hydration, and modified diet or exercise.

3. **Hypoglycemia (Low Blood Sugar):**
   - **Symptoms:** Shakiness, sweating, dizziness, confusion, hunger, rapid heartbeat.
   - **Readings:** Usually below 70 mg/dL.
   - **Action:** Treat immediately with fast-acting carbohydrates like glucose tablets,

fruit juice, or candy, and recheck blood sugar after 15 minutes.

Tips for Accurate Monitoring:

1. **Consistency:** Test at the same times each day to get a clear picture of trends and patterns.

2. **Use Reliable Equipment:** Ensure your glucose meter is calibrated and working accurately.

3. **Record Keeping:** Maintain a log of readings and note associated factors like meals, exercise, medications, and how they impact blood sugar levels.

4. **Consult Healthcare Providers:** Discuss trends or concerns with healthcare providers to adjust treatment plans as needed.

Conclusion:

Regular blood glucose monitoring empowers individuals with diabetes to take control of their condition by tracking blood sugar levels, identifying patterns, and making necessary adjustments to maintain optimal blood sugar control. Interpreting these readings and taking appropriate action based on them is crucial for effectively managing diabetes and preventing complications associated with blood sugar fluctuations.

Continuous Glucose Monitoring (CGM): Introducing CGM devices and their benefits in diabetes management:

Continuous Glucose Monitoring (CGM) devices are valuable tools used in diabetes management to provide real-time and continuous information about blood sugar levels throughout the day and night. Here's an introduction to CGM devices and their benefits:

What is Continuous Glucose Monitoring (CGM)?

1. **Continuous Monitoring:** CGM devices continuously track glucose levels in the interstitial fluid, providing readings every few minutes throughout the day and night.

2. **Sensor Technology:** Consists of a small sensor placed under the skin, usually on the abdomen, transmitting data wirelessly to a receiver or smartphone app.

3. **Data Visualization:** Offers real-time glucose readings, trends, and alerts for high or low blood sugar levels.

Benefits of CGM in Diabetes Management:

1. **Immediate Feedback:** Provides real-time glucose data, offering insights into how food, exercise, medications, and other factors affect blood sugar levels.

2. **Trend Analysis:** Displays trends and patterns, highlighting blood sugar changes throughout the day, aiding in treatment adjustments and decision-making.

3. **Hypo/Hyperglycemia Alerts:** Alerts users when blood sugar levels are trending high or low, allowing for proactive intervention to prevent severe episodes.

4. **Reduced Fingerstick Testing:** Reduces the need for frequent fingerstick tests, enhancing convenience and comfort.

5. **Improved Control:** Helps individuals and healthcare providers make informed decisions to better manage blood sugar levels and prevent extreme fluctuations.

6. **Enhanced Quality of Life:** Offers peace of mind, reducing anxiety about blood sugar fluctuations, especially during sleep or physical activity.

Considerations with CGM:

1. **Calibration:** Some CGM systems require periodic calibration with traditional fingerstick tests for accuracy.

2. **Sensor Placement:** Correct placement and adherence of the sensor are crucial for accurate readings.

3. **Cost and Insurance Coverage:** CGM devices can be expensive, and insurance coverage varies.

Conclusion:

Continuous Glucose Monitoring (CGM) devices provide real-time data on blood sugar levels, trends, and patterns, empowering individuals with diabetes to make timely adjustments in their treatment plans. The immediate feedback and alerts offered by CGM systems contribute significantly to better blood sugar control, reducing the risk of severe hypoglycemia or hyperglycemia episodes, and ultimately improving overall diabetes management and quality of life.

Tips for Effective Monitoring:** Providing practical tips for accurate blood sugar monitoring:

Absolutely! Here are some practical tips for accurate and effective blood sugar monitoring:

1. Test at Regular Intervals:

1. **Consistent Timing:** Establish a routine for testing, such as before meals, before bedtime, or as advised by healthcare providers.

2. **Post-Meal Monitoring:** Check blood sugar levels 1-2 hours after meals to understand how different foods impact blood glucose.

2. Proper Technique:

1. **Clean Hands:** Wash hands with soap and water before testing to avoid contamination affecting readings.

2. **Finger Selection:** Rotate fingers for testing to prevent soreness and ensure accurate readings.

3. Ensure Equipment Accuracy:

1. **Calibration:** Calibrate the glucose meter as recommended by the manufacturer for accurate readings.

2. **Check Strips and Meter:** Ensure strips are not expired and match the meter's coding to avoid errors.

4. Record and Analyze Readings:

1. **Keep a Log:** Maintain a blood sugar log, noting readings, time, date, meal details, medications, and activities.

2. **Identify Patterns:** Analyze trends in blood sugar levels to make informed adjustments to diet, medication, or activity.

5. Understand Target Ranges:

1. **Know Targets:** Be aware of your target blood sugar ranges set by healthcare providers for different times of the day.

2. **Interpret Results:** Understand the significance of readings to take appropriate action for high or low blood sugar levels.

6. Stay Informed and Communicate:

1. **Stay Educated:** Continuously learn about diabetes management and blood sugar monitoring through reliable sources.

2. **Consult Healthcare Providers:** Discuss trends, concerns, or changes in readings with healthcare providers for appropriate adjustments.

7. Address External Factors:

1. **Account for Influences:** Consider factors like illness, stress, medications, and menstrual cycles, which can affect blood sugar levels.

2. **Weather Impact:** Extreme temperatures can affect glucose meter performance, so store equipment properly.

8. Regular Maintenance:

1. **Meter Check-ups:** Have your glucose meter calibrated and checked regularly for accuracy.

2. **Battery and Strips:** Replace batteries and test strips as recommended by the manufacturer.

Conclusion:

Exact glucose observing is vital for compelling diabetes the board. Adhering to proper testing techniques, recording readings, understanding target ranges, and staying informed are essential for individuals to make informed decisions about their diabetes care. Regular communication with healthcare providers ensures a collaborative approach to maintaining optimal blood sugar levels and overall well-being.

Chapter 6: Coping with Diabetes - Emotional Well-being

Managing Stress:** Discussing the impact of stress on blood sugar levels and strategies to manage stress effectively.

Stress can significantly impact blood sugar levels in individuals managing diabetes. Here's an overview of its impact and strategies to effectively manage stress:

Impact of Stress on Blood Sugar Levels:

1. **Hormonal Response:** Stress triggers the release of stress hormones like cortisol and adrenaline, which can lead to increased blood sugar levels.

2. **Insulin Resistance:** Stress hormones can reduce insulin's effectiveness, leading to elevated blood sugar levels, particularly in individuals with insulin resistance.

3. **Behavioral Changes:** Stress might lead to changes in eating habits, physical activity levels, and medication adherence, all of which can affect blood sugar control.

Strategies to Manage Stress Effectively:

1. **Physical Activity:**
   - **Exercise:** Engage in regular physical activity like walking, yoga, or any preferred

form of exercise to reduce stress levels and improve blood sugar control.

2. **Relaxation Techniques:**
   - **Deep Breathing:** Practice deep breathing exercises or meditation to promote relaxation and reduce stress.

   - **Progressive Muscle Relaxation:** Tense and relax muscle groups sequentially to alleviate physical tension caused by stress.

3. **Healthy Lifestyle Choices:**
   - **Balanced Diet:** Maintain a healthy diet rich in fruits, vegetables, whole grains, and lean proteins to support overall well-being.

   - **Adequate Sleep:** Prioritize sufficient and quality sleep to reduce stress levels and support optimal blood sugar control.

4. **Stress Management Techniques:**
   - **Time Management:** Prioritize tasks and organize schedules to reduce overwhelming feelings.

   - **Mindfulness:** Practice mindfulness techniques like mindfulness meditation to increase awareness and reduce stress reactions.

5. **Seek Support:**
   - **Social Connections:** Connect with friends, family, or support groups to share feelings and receive emotional support.

   - **Professional Help:** Consider counseling or therapy to learn coping strategies and manage stress effectively.

6. **Limiting Stressors:**

- **Identify Triggers:** Recognize stressors and take steps to minimize their impact on daily life.

- **Setting Boundaries:** Establish boundaries to manage workload, relationships, or commitments.

Conclusion:

Managing stress is essential for individuals managing diabetes as it directly impacts blood sugar levels. Adopting stress management strategies like regular exercise, relaxation techniques, healthy lifestyle choices, seeking support, and effectively addressing stressors can significantly contribute to better stress management, leading to improved blood sugar control and overall well-being.

Support Systems:** Highlighting the importance of a support network and seeking professional help when needed:

Having a robust support system plays a pivotal role in managing diabetes effectively. Here's why it's crucial and the importance of seeking professional help when required:

Importance of a Support Network:

1. **Emotional Support:** Family, friends, or support groups offer understanding, empathy, and encouragement, reducing feelings of isolation or stress associated with managing diabetes.

2. **Motivation and Accountability:** Support networks provide motivation to adhere to treatment plans, maintain healthy habits, and stay consistent with blood sugar monitoring.

3. **Sharing Knowledge and Experiences:** Interacting with others who have diabetes allows for sharing experiences, tips, and coping strategies, fostering a sense of camaraderie and learning.

4. **Reduced Stress Levels:** A supportive environment can alleviate stress associated with diabetes management, positively impacting blood sugar control.

Seeking Professional Help:

1. **Healthcare Providers:** Regular communication with healthcare providers

ensures appropriate diabetes management and timely adjustments to treatment plans.

2. **Diabetes Educators:** Certified diabetes educators offer specialized knowledge, guidance, and practical advice on managing diabetes, including lifestyle modifications, medication adherence, and blood sugar monitoring.

3. **Mental Health Professionals:** Counselors, psychologists, or therapists help address emotional challenges related to diabetes, providing coping strategies and support for stress, anxiety, or depression.

4. **Nutritionists/Dietitians:** Seek guidance from professionals to create personalized meal plans and understand how diet affects blood sugar levels.

When to Seek Professional Help:

1. **Uncontrolled Blood Sugar:** If blood sugar levels consistently remain high or low despite adherence to treatment plans.

2. **Emotional Struggles:** Feelings of distress, anxiety, or depression impacting daily life or diabetes management.

3. **Difficulty Adapting:** Struggling to adhere to prescribed medications, lifestyle changes, or blood sugar monitoring.

4. **Need for Additional Guidance:** When additional information, support, or guidance is required for effective diabetes management.

Conclusion:

A strong support network comprising family, friends, healthcare providers, and diabetes educators provides invaluable assistance in managing diabetes. Seeking professional help when needed ensures comprehensive and personalized care, addressing emotional, physical, and educational needs related to diabetes management. Building and nurturing these support systems are vital for individuals to effectively navigate the challenges of living with diabetes and maintain a positive outlook on their health journey.

Embracing a Positive Mindset:** Encouraging a positive attitude towards living with diabetes:

Embracing a positive mindset while living with diabetes can significantly impact overall well-being. Here are reasons to foster a positive attitude and tips to encourage positivity:

Importance of a Positive Mindset:

1. **Empowerment:** A positive outlook empowers individuals to take charge of their health and actively manage diabetes.

2. **Reduced Stress:** Positivity helps reduce stress levels, which can positively impact blood sugar control.

3. **Adherence to Treatment:** A positive mindset encourages adherence to treatment plans, medications, blood sugar monitoring, and lifestyle modifications.

4. **Improved Resilience:** It fosters resilience, enabling individuals to cope better with challenges associated with diabetes.

Tips for Encouraging Positivity:

1. **Focus on Control, Not Perfection:** Acknowledge that managing diabetes involves effort, and progress matters more than perfection.

2. **Practice Gratitude:** Cultivate gratitude by acknowledging achievements, no matter how small, in managing diabetes.

3. **Positive Self-Talk:** Replace negative thoughts with positive affirmations and self-encouragement.

4. **Celebrate Progress:** Celebrate milestones and successes in blood sugar control or lifestyle changes.

5. **Mindfulness and Relaxation:** Engage in mindfulness exercises, meditation, or relaxation techniques to promote a calm and positive mindset.

6. **Surround Yourself with Positivity:** Surround yourself with supportive and positive influences to maintain an optimistic perspective.

7. **Seek Inspiration:** Connect with communities or individuals who inspire and motivate with their experiences in managing diabetes.

Embracing Challenges:

1. **Adaptability:** Embrace diabetes as a part of life and focus on adapting positively to changes it brings.

2. **Learning Opportunity:** View challenges as learning opportunities to improve diabetes management strategies.

3. **Maintain Perspective:** Keep a broader perspective beyond diabetes, nurturing other aspects of life like relationships, hobbies, and personal growth.

Conclusion:

Embracing a positive mindset empowers individuals to navigate the challenges of living with diabetes more effectively. By cultivating positivity through gratitude, self-encouragement, mindfulness, and celebrating successes, individuals can maintain a resilient and optimistic outlook, contributing positively to their overall well-being and successful diabetes management.

Chapter 7: Preventing Complications and Future Outlook

Complications of Diabetes:** Addressing potential complications and ways to prevent or manage them.

Certainly! Diabetes can prompt different difficulties that influence various pieces of the body. Here are some potential complications and ways to prevent or manage them:

1. Cardiovascular Complications:

1. **Prevention:** Maintain healthy blood sugar, cholesterol, and blood pressure levels through medication, diet, exercise, and regular check-ups.

2. **Management:** Follow a heart-healthy lifestyle, including a balanced diet, regular exercise, quitting smoking, and adhering to prescribed medications.

2. Neuropathy (Nerve Damage):

1. **Prevention:** Maintain stable blood sugar levels and avoid smoking.

2. **Management:** Regular foot care, monitoring for signs of neuropathy, and managing symptoms through medication or therapies as recommended by healthcare providers.

3. Nephropathy (Kidney Damage):

1. **Prevention:** Manage blood sugar and blood pressure levels, maintain a healthy weight, and limit salt intake.

2. **Management:** Regular kidney function tests, blood pressure control, medications to protect kidney function, and maintaining a kidney-friendly diet.

4. Retinopathy (Eye Damage):

1. **Prevention:** Regular eye exams, managing blood sugar and blood pressure levels, and avoiding smoking.

2. **Management:** Timely treatment with laser therapy, injections, or surgery to prevent or slow vision loss.

5. Foot Complications:

1. **Prevention:** Daily foot care, wearing proper footwear, regular foot checks, and avoiding barefoot walking.

2. **Management:** Prompt treatment of foot injuries or infections, and consulting a healthcare provider for any foot-related concerns.

6. Skin Complications:

1. **Prevention:** Keep skin clean and dry, inspect skin regularly for signs of infection or changes, and moisturize to prevent dryness.

2. **Management:** Prompt treatment of skin infections, ulcers, or wounds, and seeking medical advice for any skin changes.

Conclusion:

Preventing complications involves maintaining stable blood sugar levels, managing blood pressure and cholesterol, adopting a healthy lifestyle, and regular medical check-ups. Monitoring and addressing complications early through proper medication, lifestyle modifications, and timely medical intervention are crucial in managing diabetes and minimizing the impact of potential complications on overall health and well-being. Regular communication with healthcare providers is essential to identify and address any emerging complications effectively.

Living a Fulfilling Life:** Offering guidance on leading a fulfilling life while managing diabetes:

Absolutely! Managing diabetes doesn't have to limit one's ability to lead a fulfilling life. Here's guidance on living life to the fullest while managing diabetes:

1. Embrace Self-Care:

1. **Prioritize Health:** Make self-care a priority by managing blood sugar, eating a balanced diet, exercising regularly, and taking prescribed medications.

2. **Mindfulness Practices:** Engage in mindfulness, meditation, or relaxation

techniques to reduce stress and enhance overall well-being.

2. Maintain a Positive Mindset:

1. **Focus on Positivity:** Cultivate a positive outlook by celebrating achievements, practicing gratitude, and engaging in activities that bring joy.

2. **Community Engagement:** Connect with supportive communities or groups that share similar experiences, fostering a sense of belonging and encouragement.

3. Pursue Hobbies and Passions:

1. **Explore Interests:** Pursue hobbies, interests, or activities that bring happiness and fulfillment, ensuring diabetes management integrates seamlessly into life.

2. **Physical Activities:** Engage in physical activities that are enjoyable, promoting both physical and mental well-being.

4. **Strong Support System:**

1. **Family and Friends:** Build a supportive network of family and friends who understand and encourage diabetes management.

2. **Healthcare Team:** Foster a strong relationship with healthcare providers for guidance, support, and regular monitoring.

5. **Set and Pursue Goals:**

1. **Personal Development:** Set achievable goals related to career, education, personal growth, or hobbies.

2. **Health Goals:** Establish realistic health goals, monitor progress, and celebrate achievements in diabetes management.

6. Educate and Advocate:

1. **Continuous Learning:** Stay informed about diabetes through reliable sources, attending workshops, or seeking information from healthcare providers.

2. **Advocacy:** Consider becoming an advocate for diabetes awareness, sharing experiences, and supporting others in their journey.

Conclusion:

Living a fulfilling life while managing diabetes involves embracing self-care, maintaining a positive mindset, pursuing interests and hobbies, building a strong support network, setting and pursuing meaningful goals, and continually educating oneself about diabetes. With proactive diabetes management and a holistic approach to life, individuals can lead fulfilling and vibrant lives, ensuring diabetes doesn't hinder their pursuit of happiness and success.

Future of Diabetes Management: Exploring advancements and potential breakthroughs in diabetes treatment:**

Absolutely! The future of diabetes management holds promise with ongoing research and advancements in treatment. Here are some areas of potential breakthroughs and advancements:

1. Continuous Glucose Monitoring (CGM) and Insulin Delivery:

1. **Closed-Loop Systems:** Enhancements in closed-loop insulin delivery systems (artificial pancreas) that automatically adjust insulin based on real-time CGM data, reducing the need for manual intervention.

2. **Implantable Devices:** Development of implantable or long-acting devices for continuous insulin delivery, offering convenience and improving adherence to treatment.

2. Advanced Medications and Therapies:

1. **New Insulin Formulations:** Ultra-rapid and more stable insulins with faster onset and shorter duration, allowing for

better control and flexibility in insulin delivery.

2. **Targeted Therapies:** Advancements in medications targeting specific pathways to improve blood sugar control with fewer side effects.

3. Personalized Medicine:

1. **Precision Medicine:** Tailoring treatment plans based on an individual's genetic, metabolic, and lifestyle factors for more personalized and effective diabetes management.

2. **Predictive Analytics:** Utilizing artificial intelligence and predictive models to foresee blood sugar trends and prevent hyper/hypoglycemic events before they occur.

4. **Regenerative Therapies:**

1. **Beta Cell Regeneration:** Research into regenerative therapies to restore or regenerate pancreatic beta cells responsible for insulin production.

2. **Stem Cell Therapy:** Investigating the potential of stem cell therapy to regenerate insulin-producing cells or enhance insulin sensitivity.

5. **Digital Health Technologies:**

1. **Mobile Apps and Telemedicine:** Advancements in mobile applications and telemedicine to facilitate remote monitoring, virtual consultations, and personalized diabetes management.

2. **Wearable Sensors:** Integration of wearable sensors for real-time health data collection, aiding in better management and immediate interventions.

Conclusion:

The future of diabetes management holds exciting possibilities, including advancements in continuous monitoring, innovative medications and therapies, personalized treatment approaches, regenerative therapies, and the integration of digital health technologies. These breakthroughs aim to offer more precise, convenient, and effective diabetes management, ultimately improving the quality of life for individuals living with diabetes. Continued research and development pave the way for a brighter future in diabetes care.

Conclusion:Empowering Diabetes Management

Summary of Key Rules: Summarizing key takeaways from the book.**

Absolutely, summarizing the key rules or takeaways from the book "The Total Diabetes Rules":

1. Commitment to Self-Care:

- Prioritize self-care by managing blood sugar levels, adhering to medications, maintaining a balanced diet, and engaging in regular physical activity.

2. Knowledge is Empowerment:

- Teach yourself about diabetes, its administration, and likely intricacies. Knowledge empowers better decision-making and effective self-management.

3. **Blood Sugar Monitoring:**

- Regularly monitor blood sugar levels to understand patterns, identify trends, and make necessary adjustments in treatment plans and lifestyle.

4. **Healthy Lifestyle Habits:**

- Embrace a healthy lifestyle with a balanced diet, regular exercise, stress management, adequate sleep, and avoidance of harmful habits like smoking.

5. **Support and Professional Guidance:**

- Build a strong support system with family, friends, and healthcare providers for encouragement, advice, and guidance in managing diabetes.

6. **Positive Mindset:**

- Foster a positive attitude, celebrate small victories, and maintain optimism to navigate challenges associated with diabetes effectively.

7. **Continuous Learning and Adaptation:**

- Embrace continuous learning, stay updated with advancements in diabetes care, adapt to changes, and adopt personalized strategies for effective diabetes management.

8. **Future of Diabetes Management:**

- Explore and stay informed about advancements in diabetes technology, treatments, and potential breakthroughs for better management and improved quality of life.

Conclusion:

"The Total Diabetes Rules" emphasizes the importance of self-care, knowledge, regular monitoring, healthy habits, support, positivity, adaptability, and staying informed about advancements in diabetes care. By following these rules, individuals can effectively manage diabetes, minimize complications, and lead fulfilling lives.

Encouragement and Motivation:** Inspiring readers to take charge of their health and diabetes management:

Absolutely! Here's some encouragement and motivation to inspire readers to take charge of their health and diabetes management:

You're in Control:

- Your daily choices impact your health. Embrace the power you have in managing your diabetes. Every positive step you take adds up to a healthier future.

Progress, Not Perfection:

- There's no need to focus on being awesome, yet about progress. Celebrate every small victory – managing blood sugar, adopting healthier habits, or seeking support.

Empower Yourself:

- Knowledge is your best tool. Educate yourself about diabetes. Understanding empowers you to make informed decisions and take control of your health.

You're Not Alone:

- You're part of a community. Seek support, share experiences, and learn from others. Your journey with diabetes is unique, but many share similar experiences.

Challenges Lead to Growth:

- Every challenge is an opportunity for growth. Overcoming obstacles in diabetes management makes you stronger and more resilient.

Your Health, Your Priority:

- Your health is invaluable. Prioritize self-care – manage stress, eat well, exercise, and stick to your treatment plan. Putting resources into your wellbeing delivers long lasting profits.

Believe in Yourself:

- You're capable of managing diabetes effectively. Have confidence in your ability to make positive changes and live a fulfilling life despite diabetes.

Conclusion:

You have the strength, resilience, and support to navigate life with diabetes. Embrace the journey, be proactive in your health, and remember that every step towards better management counts. You're in control of your health, and your efforts will make a significant difference in leading a healthy and fulfilling life with diabetes.

REVIEW REQUEST

Dear Reader,

Thank you for exploring the pages of "Eat Right and Stay Alive: A fantastic low cholesterol cookbook and all you need to know to save your life" by Flora S. Trevino.

We strive to continuously improve and provide our readers with valuable insights into heart-healthy eating. Your feedback and reviews are incredibly valuable in guiding us on this journey.

If you've enjoyed exploring the recipes and insights within this book, we kindly invite you to share your thoughts and experiences by leaving a review. Your feedback can inspire others to embark on

their own path to a healthier lifestyle and culinary adventure.

Your honest review can help spread awareness about the transformative power of mindful, heart-conscious eating and the efforts behind creating this culinary masterpiece.

Thank you for being a part of our journey toward healthier living.

Warm regards,
Flora S. Trevino.

www.ingramcontent.com/pod-product-compliance
Lightning Source LLC
Chambersburg PA
CBHW070852260726
48661CB00004B/1369